The Beginner's Guide to the *Pegan Diet*

Ron Kness

Published by:

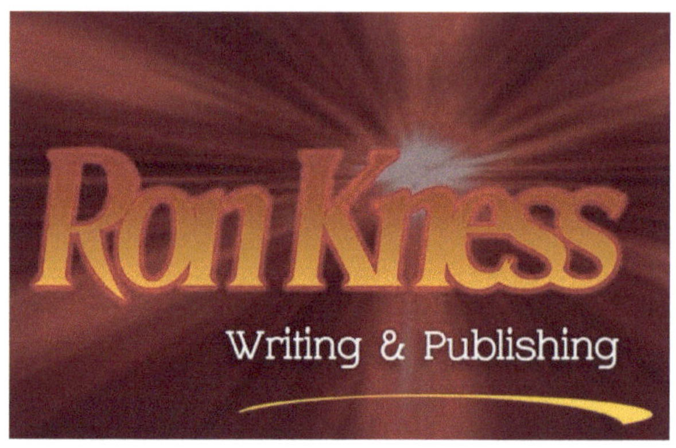

https://ronknesswriting.com

Ron Kness

Queen Creek, AZ

United States of America

For

Healthy Lifestyle Newsletter

https://healthylifestylenewsletter.com

ISBN: 9798656526685

Disclaimer

This publication is for informational purposes only and is not intended as medical advice. Medical advice should always be obtained from a qualified medical professional for any health conditions or symptoms associated with them.

Every possible effort has been made in preparing and researching this material. We make no warranties with respect to the accuracy, applicability of its contents or any omissions.

See your healthcare professional before starting any diet, health or exercise program!

Contents

What is the Pegan Diet?

When you're looking to lose weight or just generally get healthier, you'll find a lot of diet plans you can follow. One of the latest combines two of the most popular diets in recent times – Paleo and veganism.

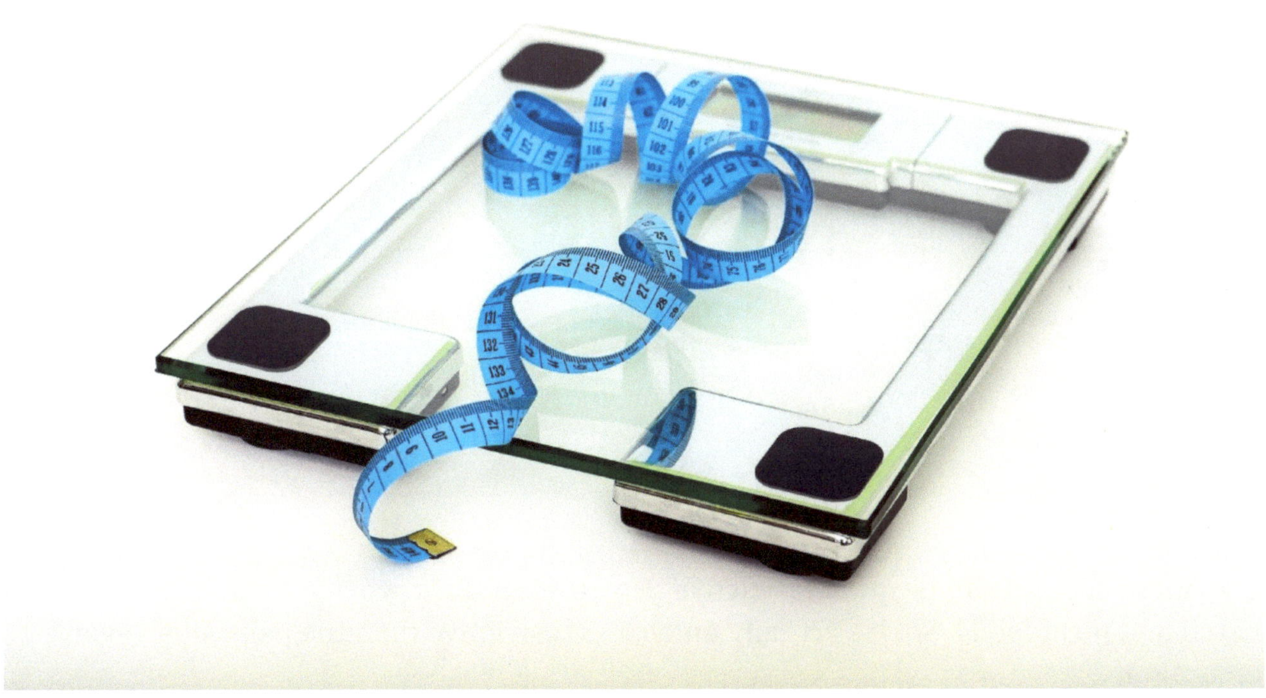

The Pegan diet is quickly becoming a popular diet option. So, what exactly is it and how does it work? Below, you'll discover everything you need to know.

What is the Pegan diet?

The Pegan diet was developed by Dr. Mark Hymen. While it is only just starting to gain traction, the diet was actually created back in 2014.

The diet is dubbed a clean, healthy eating plan and is said to deliver a lot of awesome health benefits. Dr. Hymen hasn't released any official books about the diet, though he does talk about it at length on his website.

It was developed based on the theory that whole, nutrient-rich foods can balance out the blood sugar and reduce inflammation. It's more of a long-term diet which aims to become part of your everyday lifestyle.

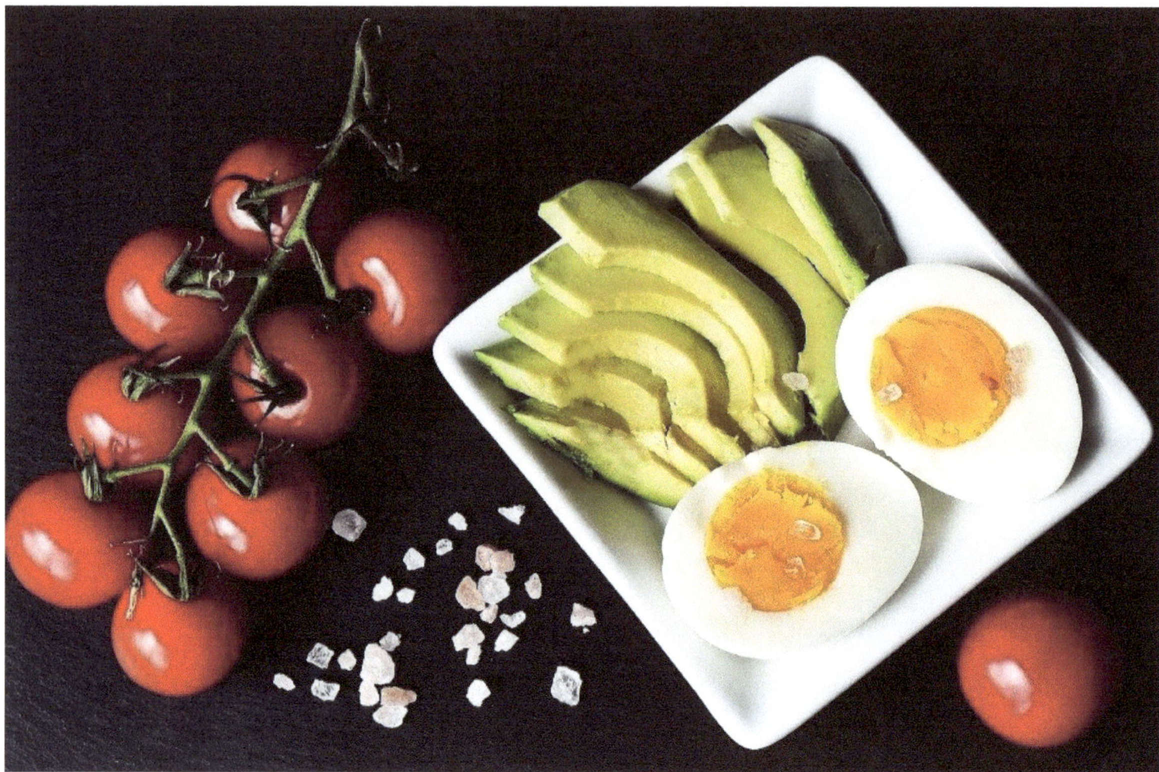

Like many diets, it can be quite restrictive. However, it does provide a mixture of plant-based and meat foods. So, it's actually much less restrictive than the paleo and vegan diets alone.

How does it work?

The good news about this diet is that it doesn't provide strict rules over what you should eat for each meal. Instead, it provides you with more of an outline that you can follow.

There are basic principles listed that you'll need to stick to if you want the diet to be successful. Some food groups are restricted, and others should be consumed in moderation.

The main rule is to try and make your diet 75% plant-based and 25% animal-based. It also focuses on gluten-free foods, although not for the reasons you'd expect. The main reason gluten is restricted from the diet with this plan, is because grains weren't considered a part of the caveman diet (crucial for followers of the Paleo diet).

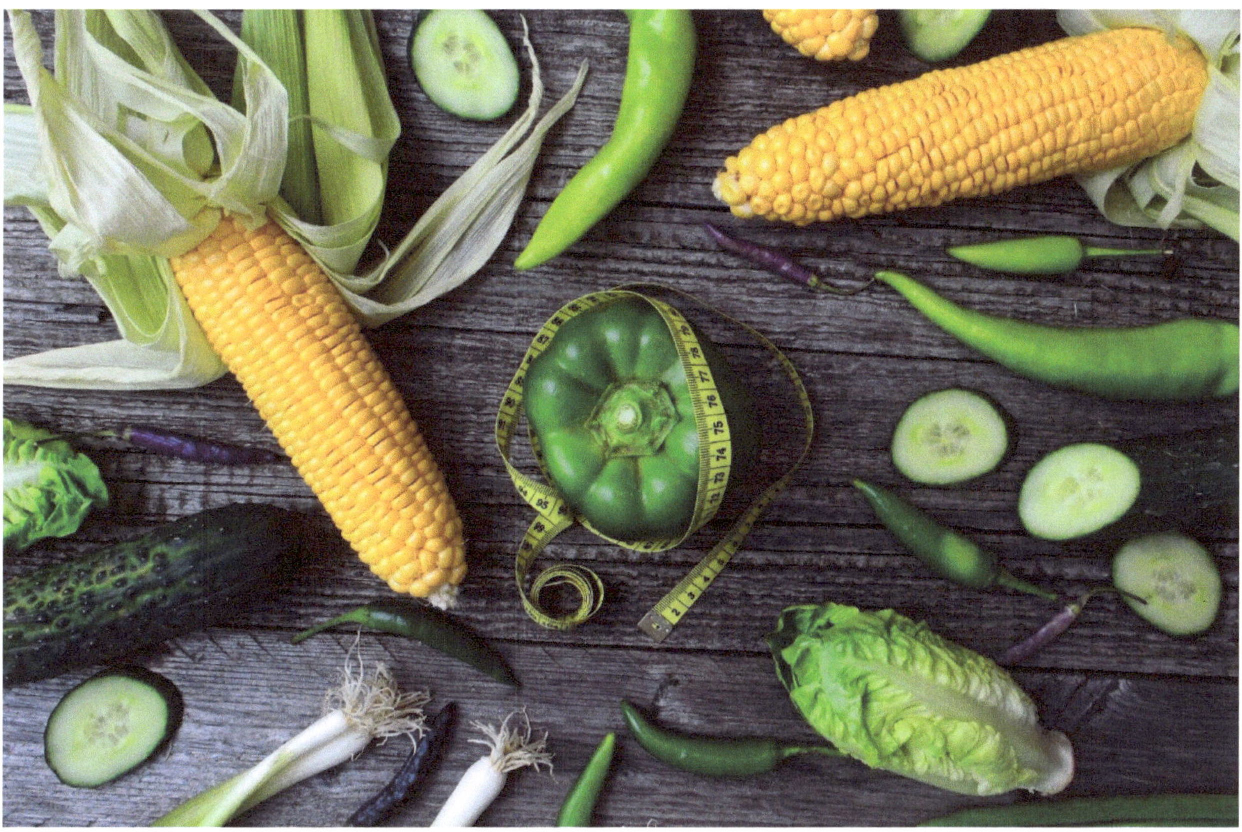

Potential challenges of the diet

While the Pegan diet is said to deliver a lot of great benefits, there are some challenges to maintaining this diet plan.

If you're using it to lose weight, you may find that it can be quite tough to follow all of the restrictions in place. Compared to many other weight loss diets, it will take a lot more effort.

As sugar is eliminated, you may also find it really hard to stick to. Obviously, a sugar-free diet is considered healthier. However, the trouble is if you cut out anything from your diet, your body is going to want it. So, resisting the cravings can be extremely difficult, particularly if your previous diet was high in sugar.

Other potential challenges include knowing what you can eat when you're out with friends, as well as coming up with meal ideas at home. The entire dairy group is eliminated so these restrictions can be difficult to navigate when looking for suitable recipes.

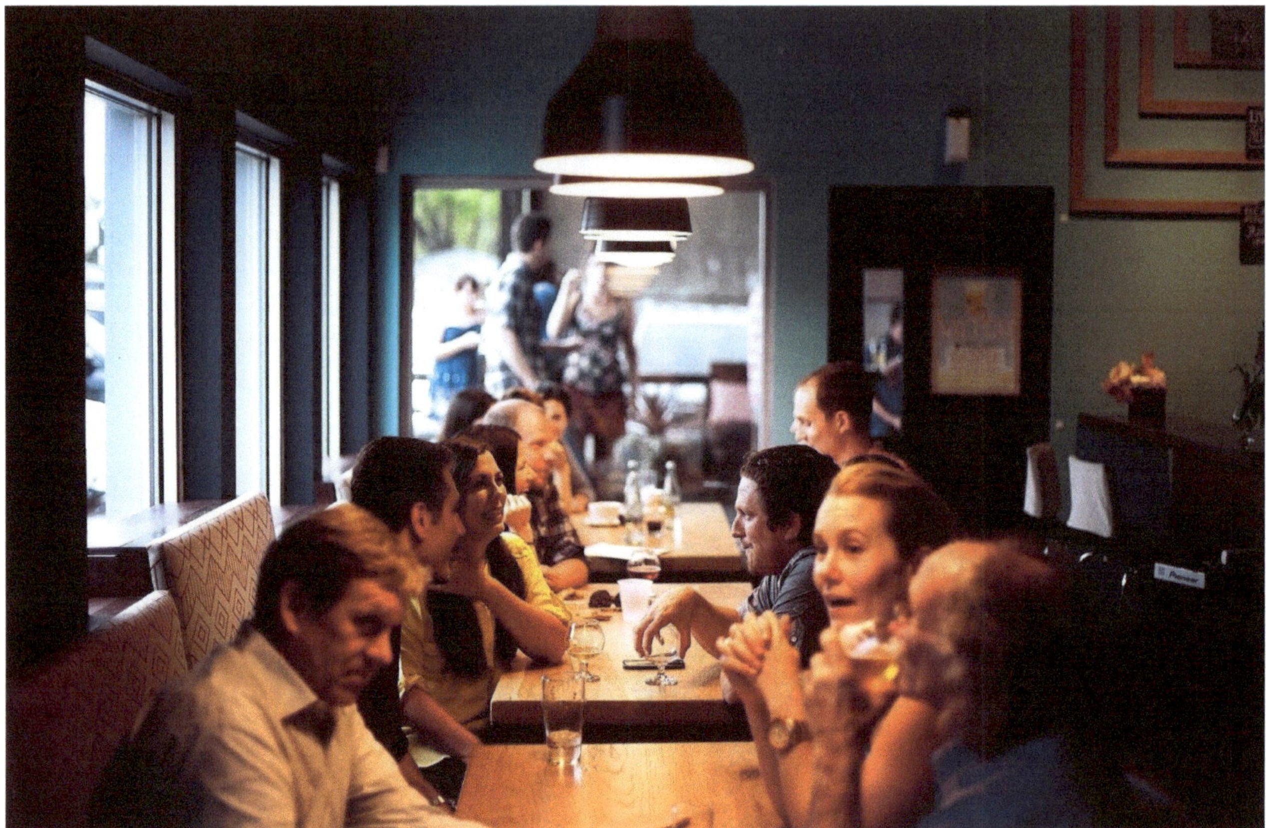

Even when you can decide what you're going to eat, you'll end up spending a lot more time in the kitchen. This isn't a bad thing, but it can be difficult for those who struggle with time management. It also means that this diet is going to be a little more expensive to follow which might not be ideal for those on a budget.

The above is just a brief overview of the Pegan diet. Now that you know what it is and how it works, it's time to research more into the basic principles of the diet. Once you have a good understanding of those, you can decide whether or not this diet is right for you.

The Basics of the Pegan Diet

The Pegan diet combines elements from both the vegan and paleo diets. However, before you decide whether or not this is the right diet plan for you, it's important to carry out a little research.

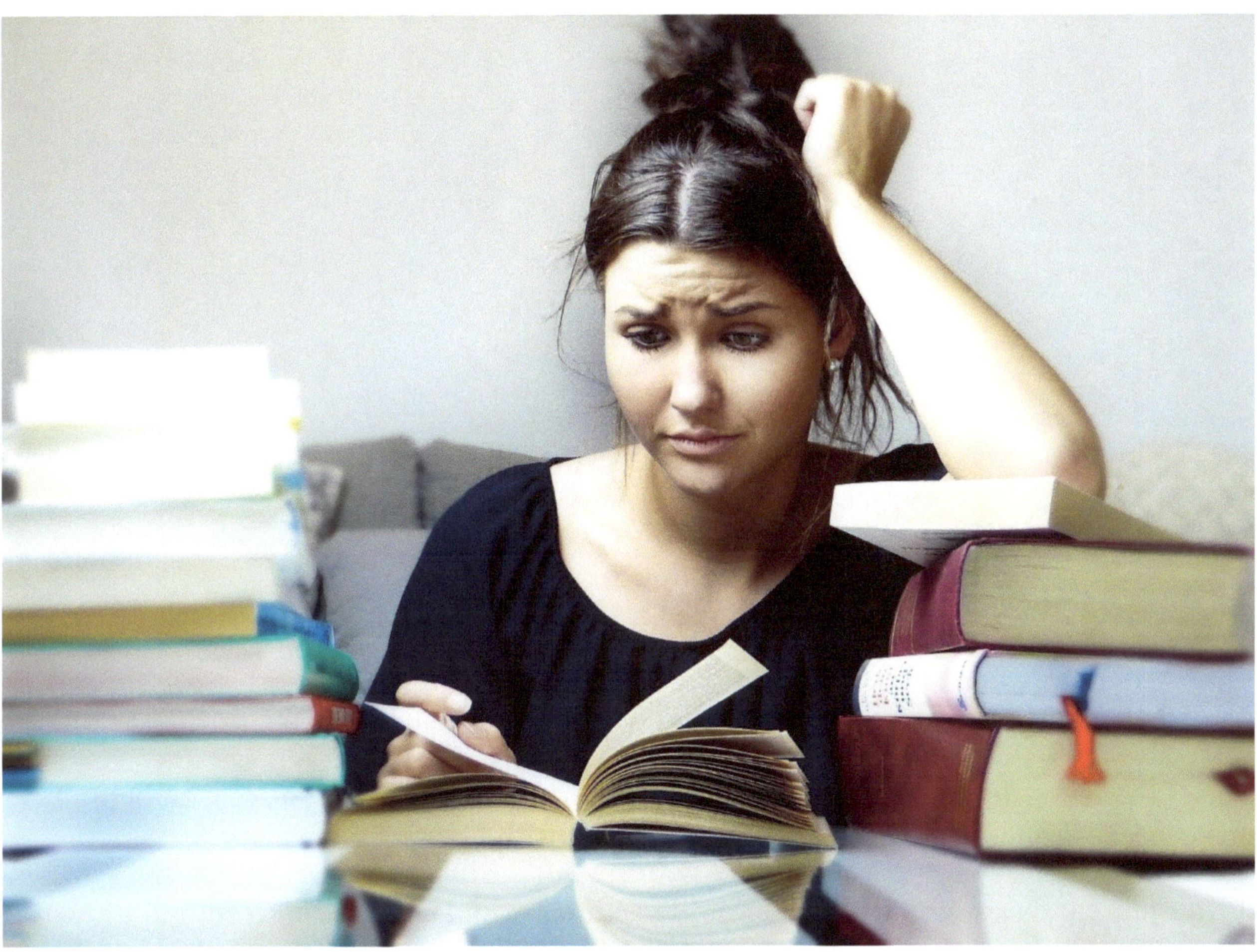

Here, you'll discover some of the basics of the Pegan diet. If you want to get the best results from this diet plan, you'll want to make sure you follow these basic rules.

Focus more on plant-based foods

The majority of the Pegan diet centers around plant-based foods. You should try to ensure your daily diet consists of around 75% plant-based foods.

You'll want to aim for a variety of vegetables and fruits. However, when it comes to fruit, try to limit your intake to low-glycemic fruits such as kiwis, berries and watermelon. Dried fruits should be avoided, and grapes and bananas should be limited.

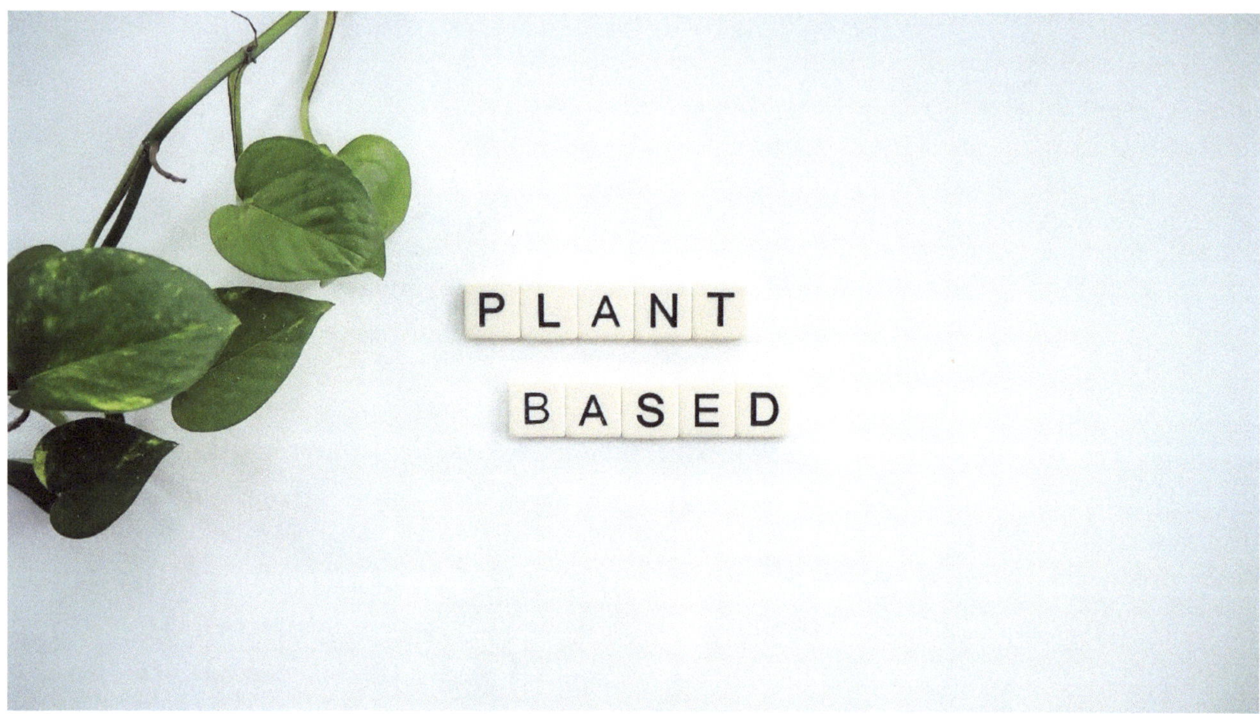

Avoid the sugar

One of the few strict restrictions on this diet, is to eliminate sugar. The reason behind this is because sugary foods can play havoc with insulin production.

It isn't just candy and sugary drinks you'll need to avoid. Don't forget to cut out hidden sugar foods such as flour and refined carbohydrates, along with foods that have added sugar.

While it does tell you to avoid sugar, you can still have it as a very occasional treat.

Consume healthier fats

Although fats get a bad rep, some of them are actually good for us. With the Pegan diet you'll want to stick to healthier fats such as Omega 3 fatty acids.

You can also consume saturated fats in moderation, provided they come from eggs, grass-fed meat and virgin coconut oil for example.

Eat plenty of seeds and nuts

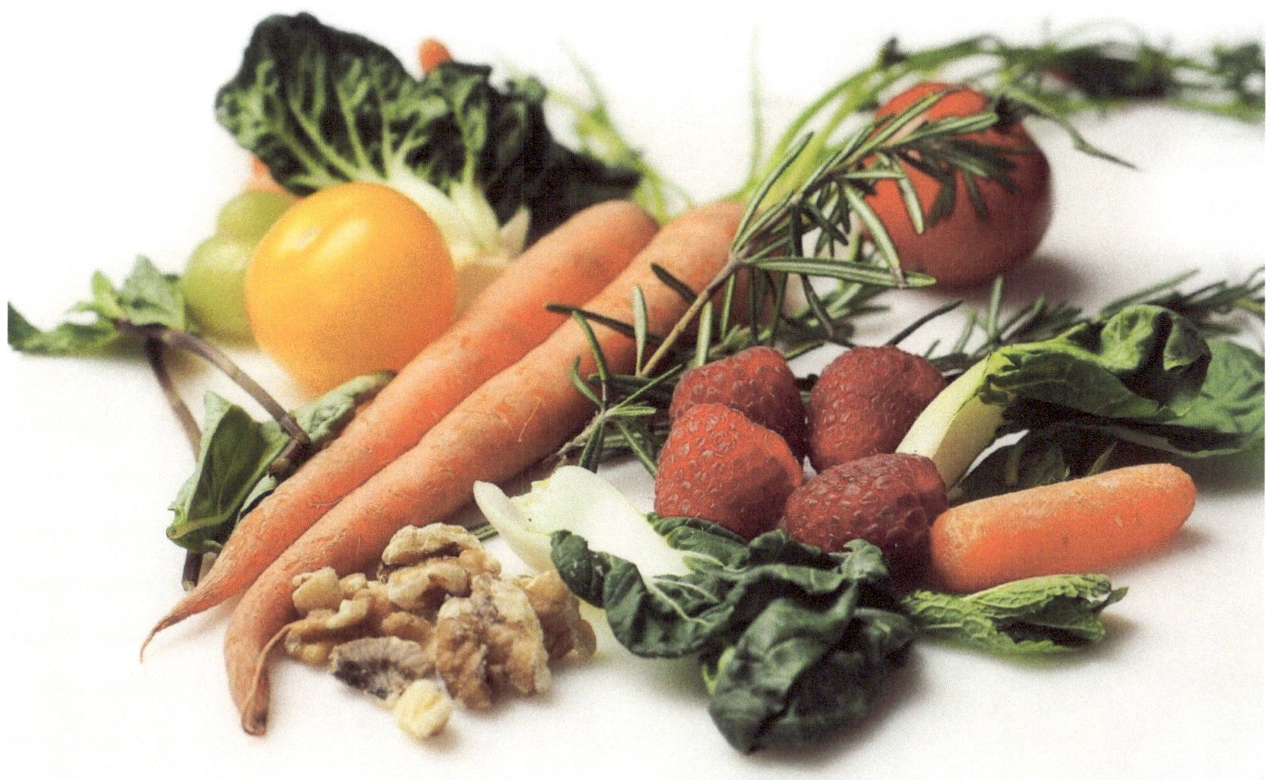

To avoid getting hungry between meals, you can snack on seeds and nuts. These provide an excellent source of protein, fiber and Omega 3 fats. It can be difficult getting the nutrients you need with a largely plant-based diet. However, nuts and seeds contain a high level of micronutrients.

Avoid pesticides, chemicals and additives

One of the key principles of this diet, is that the foods you eat should be whole and clean. This means, they can't have been grown or produced using pesticides, chemicals or additives.

The general rule is, if you can't find an ingredient in your pantry, don't put it into your body.

Eat gluten free foods

Another basic principle of this diet is to avoid foods that contain gluten. This basically includes all grain-based products made from wheat, barley, bulgar, oats and rye. This is great news for those who already follow a gluten free diet, as well as for those who are looking to eliminate it from their diets. Corn, millet, rice and sorghum are all gluten-free.

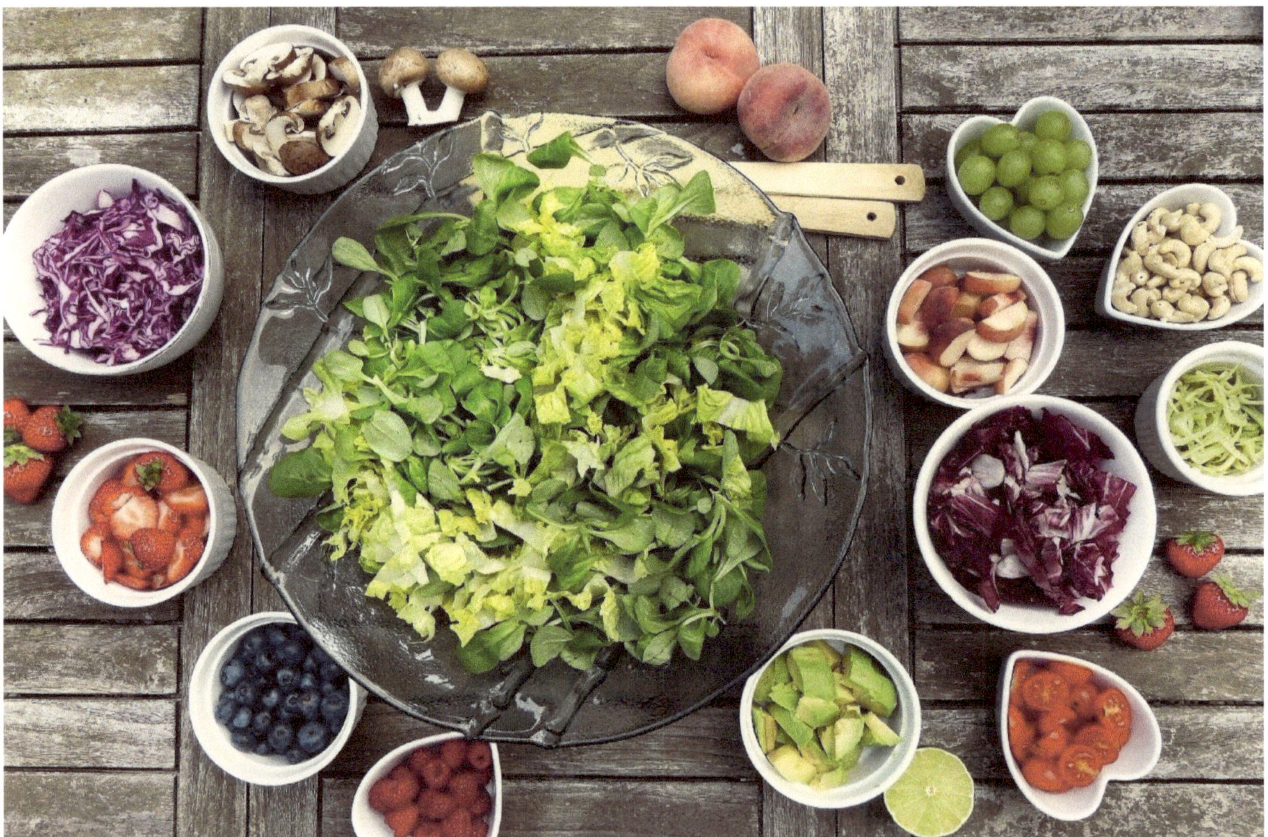

Wholegrains and legumes

The only type of grains you can occasionally eat here are wholegrains. They should still be eaten in moderation, however. Just make sure you serve up small portions at a time and opt for grains such as quinoa or black rice.

You'll also want to take it easy on the legumes. The majority of legumes are restricted from the diet due to their ability to cause issues with blood sugar. The only type of legumes you may eat occasionally include lentils.

Avoid dairy

Dairy should be restricted on a Pegan diet. However, if you find it too difficult to cut it out completely, you can use it sparingly in your diet. You can also swap cow dairy products for sheep or goat products as these aren't as bad for the body.

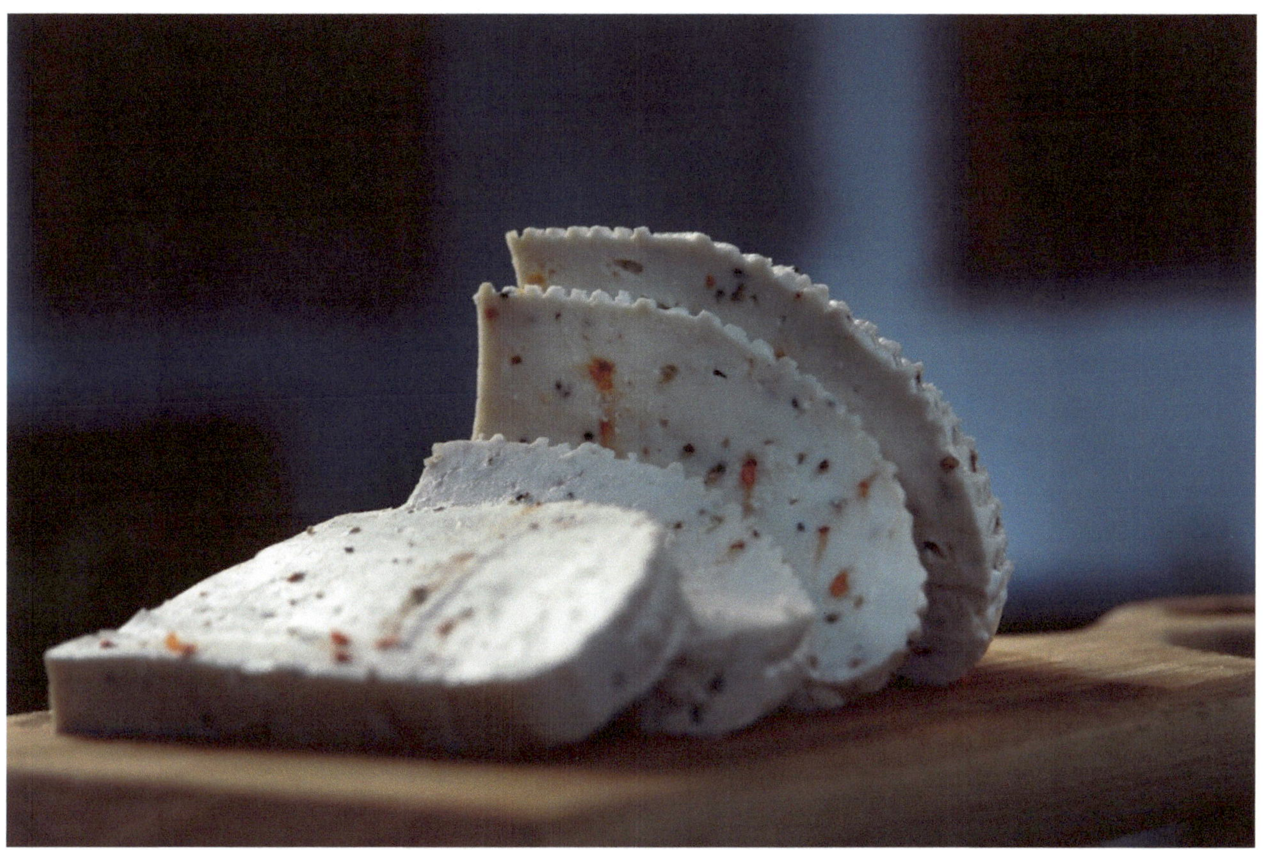

These are the main basic rules you'll need to know if you're starting the Pegan diet. As you can see, there are some restrictions. However, compared to a lot of other diets out there, you still get a good variety of foods.

List of Pegan Diet Foods

Although the Pegan diet isn't as restrictive as the Paleo or vegan diet alone, it can still be quite challenging figuring out what you can eat.

Here, we'll look at a list of Pegan diet foods you can consume. This should give you a good idea of what to expect from the diet and provide inspiration for getting started.

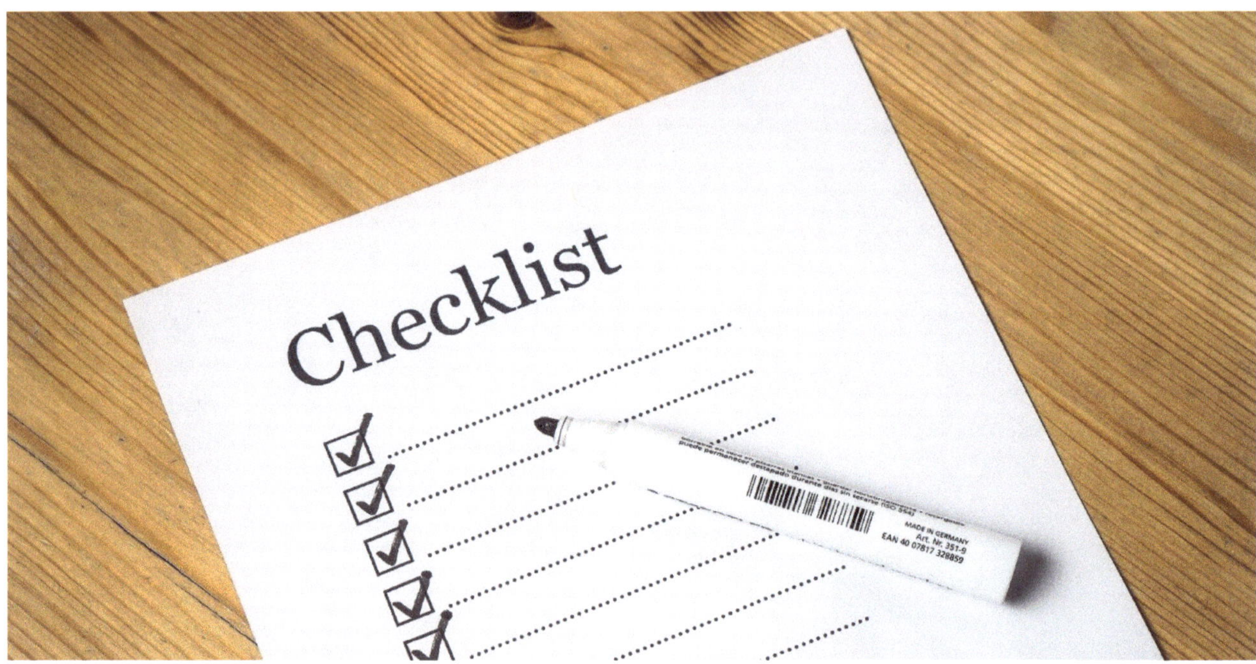

What can you eat?

So, what types of foods can you eat on the Pegan diet? The main list includes:

- Vegetables and fruits
- Seeds and nuts
- Meat
- Fish
- Eggs
- Some types of oils

The majority of the diet should be made up of vegetables, while meats should be considered more of a side dish.

Plant-based foods

When choosing your plant-based foods, it's important to limit starchy vegetables. Instead, opt for low-glycemic veggies, such as broccoli, brussels sprouts, mushrooms and cauliflower.

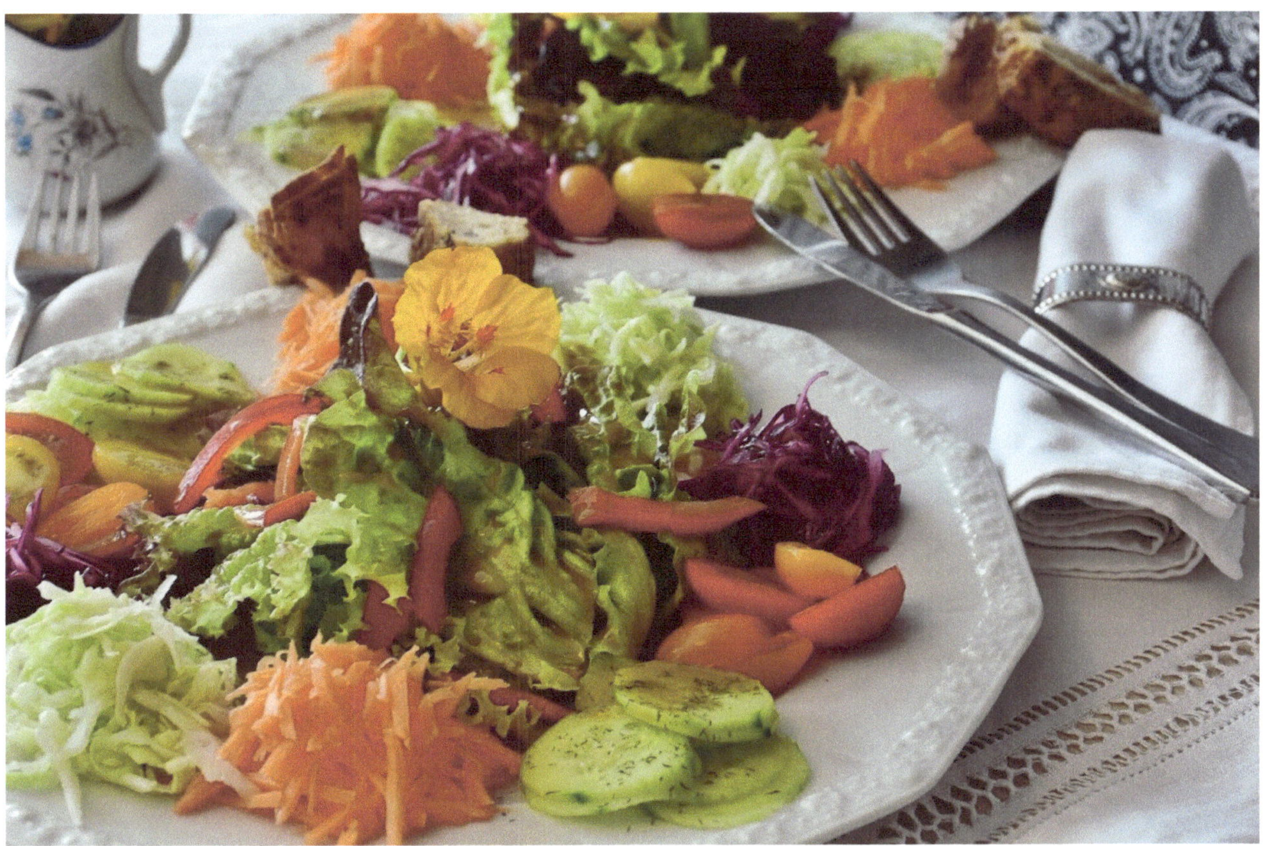

The bulk of your calorie intake will come from these veggies. That's why the Pegan diet is often considered great for weight loss.

The fruits you can eat are also limited to low-glycemic options. This is because a lot of fruits can be high in natural sugars which can cause the blood sugar levels to spike. Some of the best fruits to add to your shopping list include apples, citrus fruits, cherries and pineapple.

However, there are no strict limitations here, you can eat all types of fruits and vegetables on the diet, it's just better to choose ones with a low-glycemic index.

Seeds and nuts

It can be a real struggle to get the nutrients you need from a largely plant-based diet. That's why it is recommended you snack on seeds and nuts when following the Pegan diet.

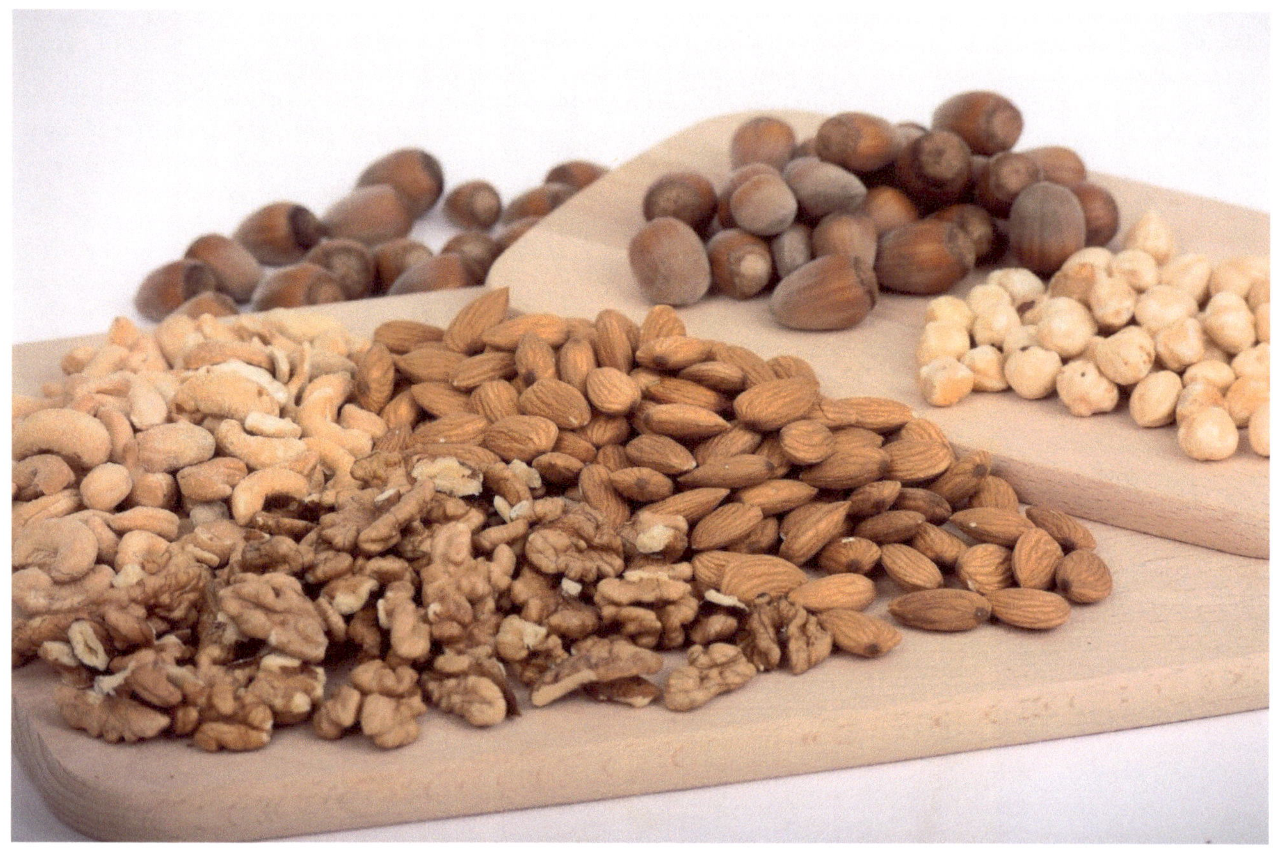

As well as providing you with the nutrients you need to stay healthy, they will also provide a good level of protein and fiber. This can really help with the digestive tract, ensuring you don't end up suffering with issues such as constipation.

Nuts and seeds can also help you to stay fuller for longer, ensuring you aren't as tempted to cheat on the diet. One of the key challenges of dieting is finding yourself constantly hungry. So, by snacking on nuts and seeds you'll stay satisfied while delivering great nutrients to the body.

Animal products

You can also eat animal products on the Pegan diet, though you'll be eating them in very small quantities.

You're also going to need to focus on grass-fed meats such as lamb and beef. Interestingly, the diet also recommends more unusual meats such as Bison and Ostrich. If you struggle to find grass-fed meat, you can also focus on sustainably raised, locally sourced meats.

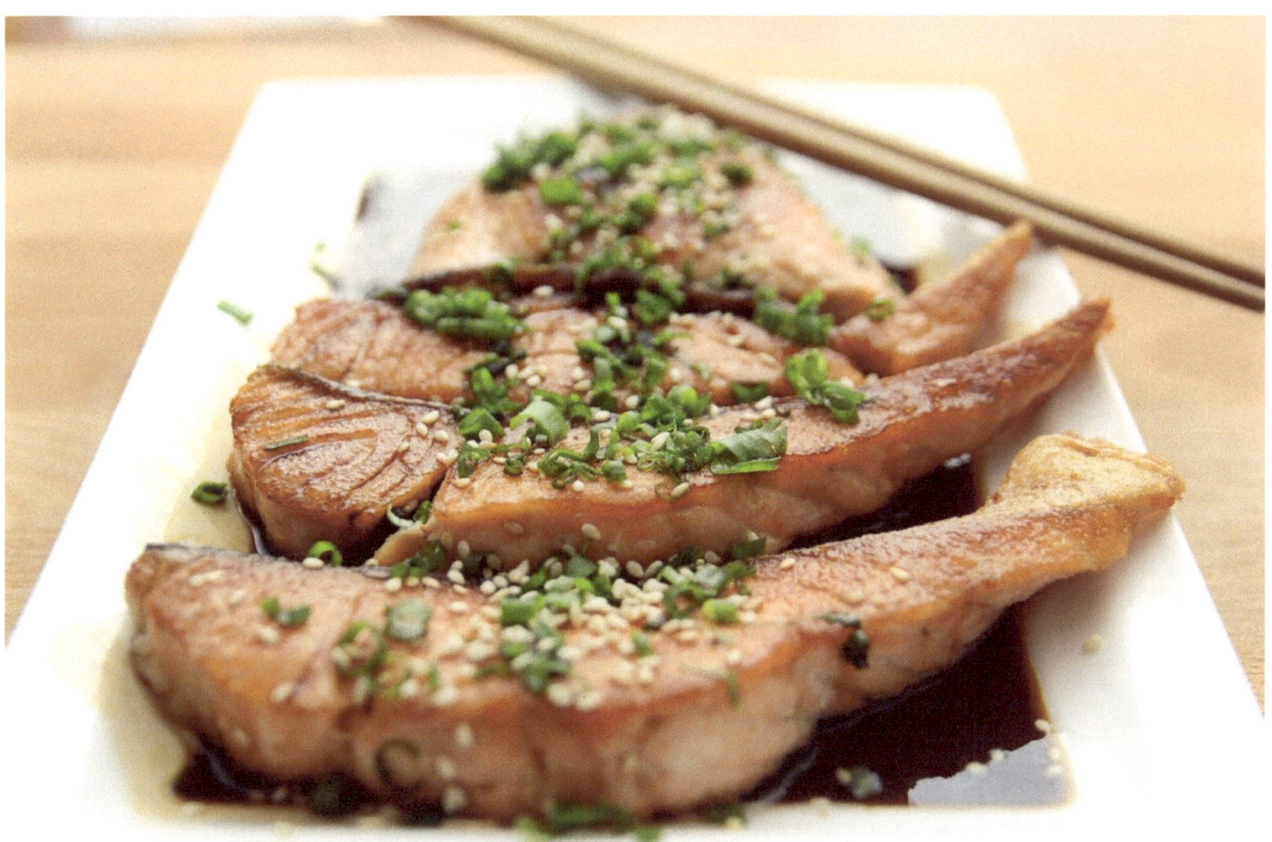

Fish is another thing you can eat. The creator of the diet recommends sticking to low-mercury fish such as sardines. However, the occasional salmon is also good as it contains high levels of Omega 3 fatty acids.

Other things you can eat sparingly

As well as the foods listed above, there are some others you can eat on a more sparingly basis.

Legumes tend to be advised against, though they can be eaten in moderation. In particular, you can eat small amounts of beans as they are a great source of fiber.

You can also minimize your consumption of natural sugars such as maple syrup, dates, honey and coconut sugar.

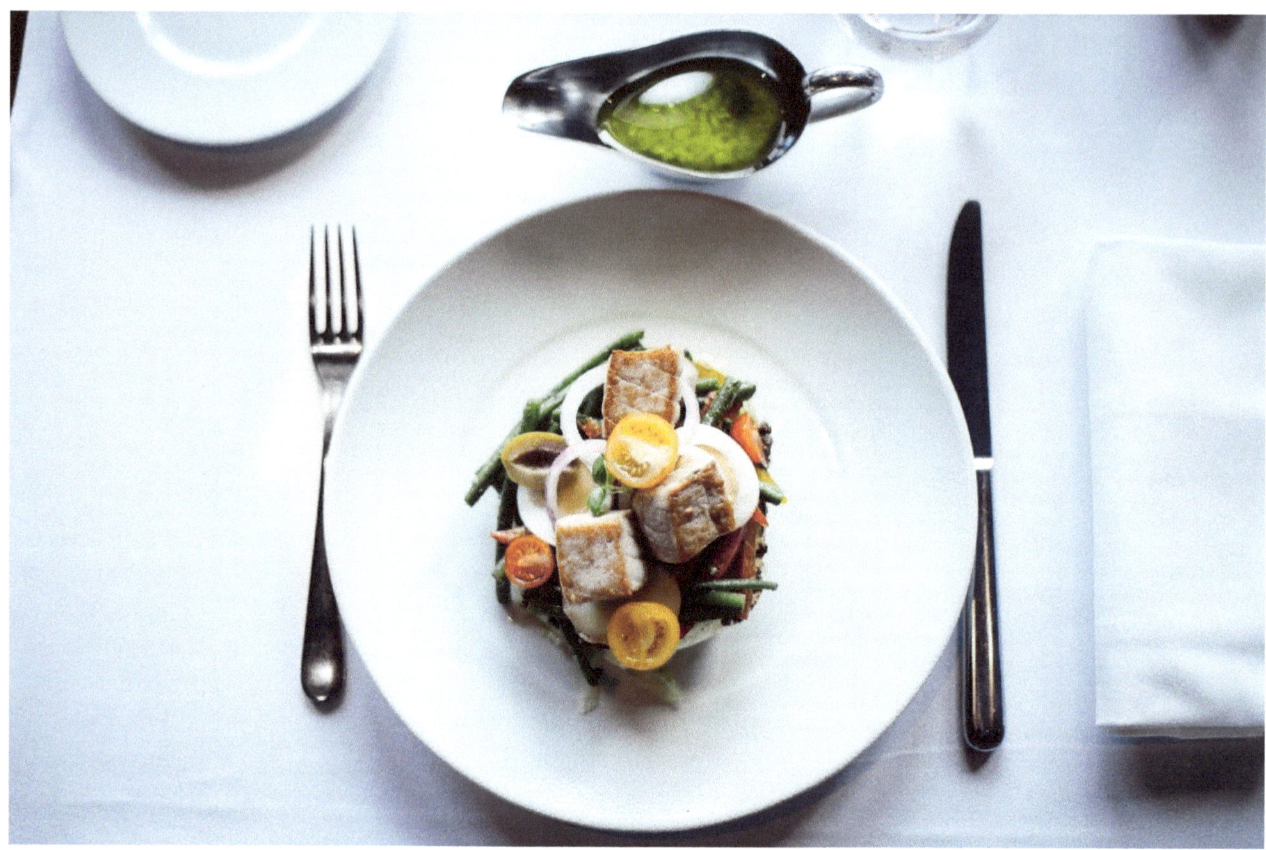

These are the main foods you can eat on the Pegan diet. While some of the recommended foods, such as Bison, aren't easy to find, the majority should be available locally. You'll need a list of these foods handy, especially when you're just getting started with the diet. Having a list of foods you can eat will make shopping for the diet a lot easier.

Pegan Foods to Avoid

As well understanding the foods you can eat on the Pegan diet, it's also important to understand the foods you'll need to avoid.

While it definitely isn't as restrictive as a lot of other diets, there are still some definite foods you can't include in this diet. Here, we'll take a look at the Pegan foods you'll want to avoid.

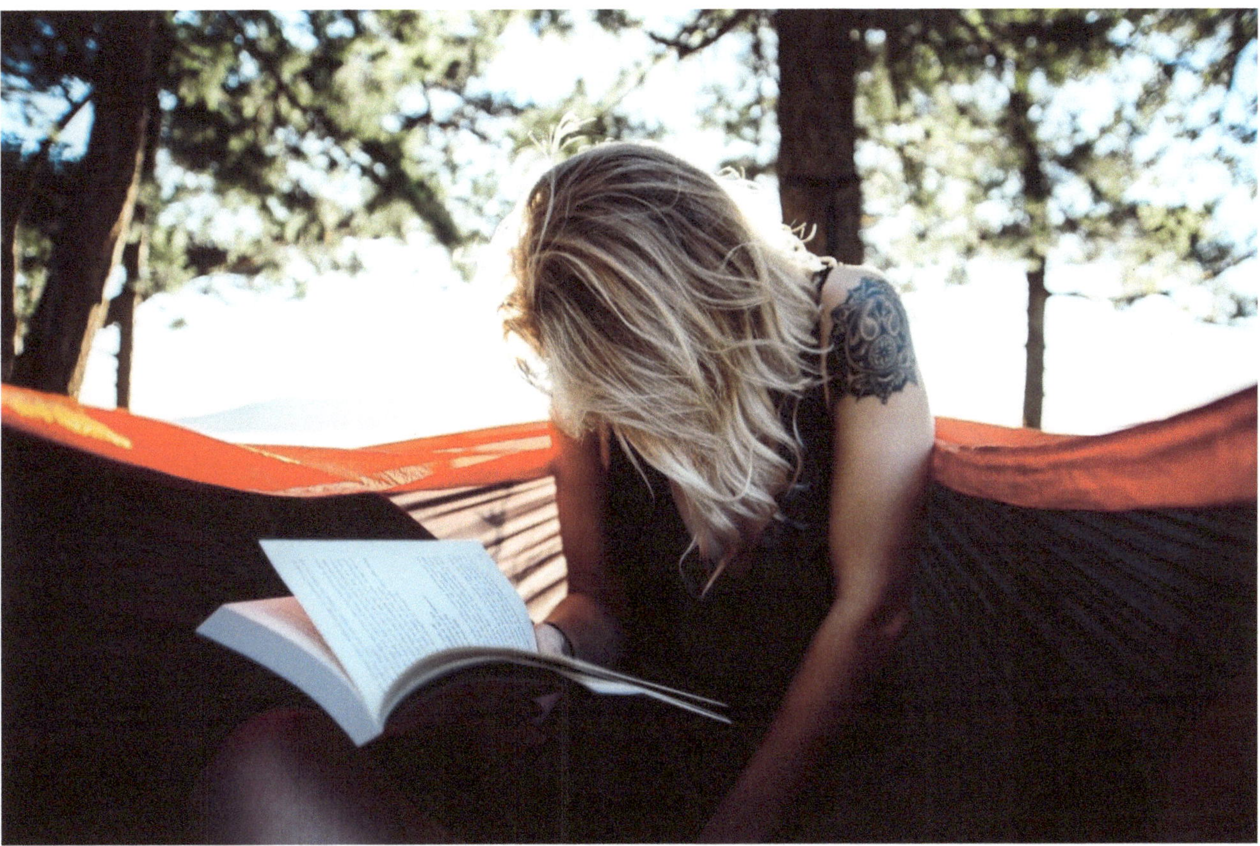

Dairy

Although the main rule is to avoid any type of dairy, you could always limit it if you don't want to cut it out completely.

The main reason this food group is restricted from the diet is because its creator believes it leads to obesity and serious diseases such as cancer.

The main types of dairy to avoid include:

- Milk
- Yoghurt
- Butter
- Cheese

It's also worth noting here that it is largely cow's milk and dairy products that are restricted. If you stick to goat or sheep dairy products, they can be eaten in small quantities.

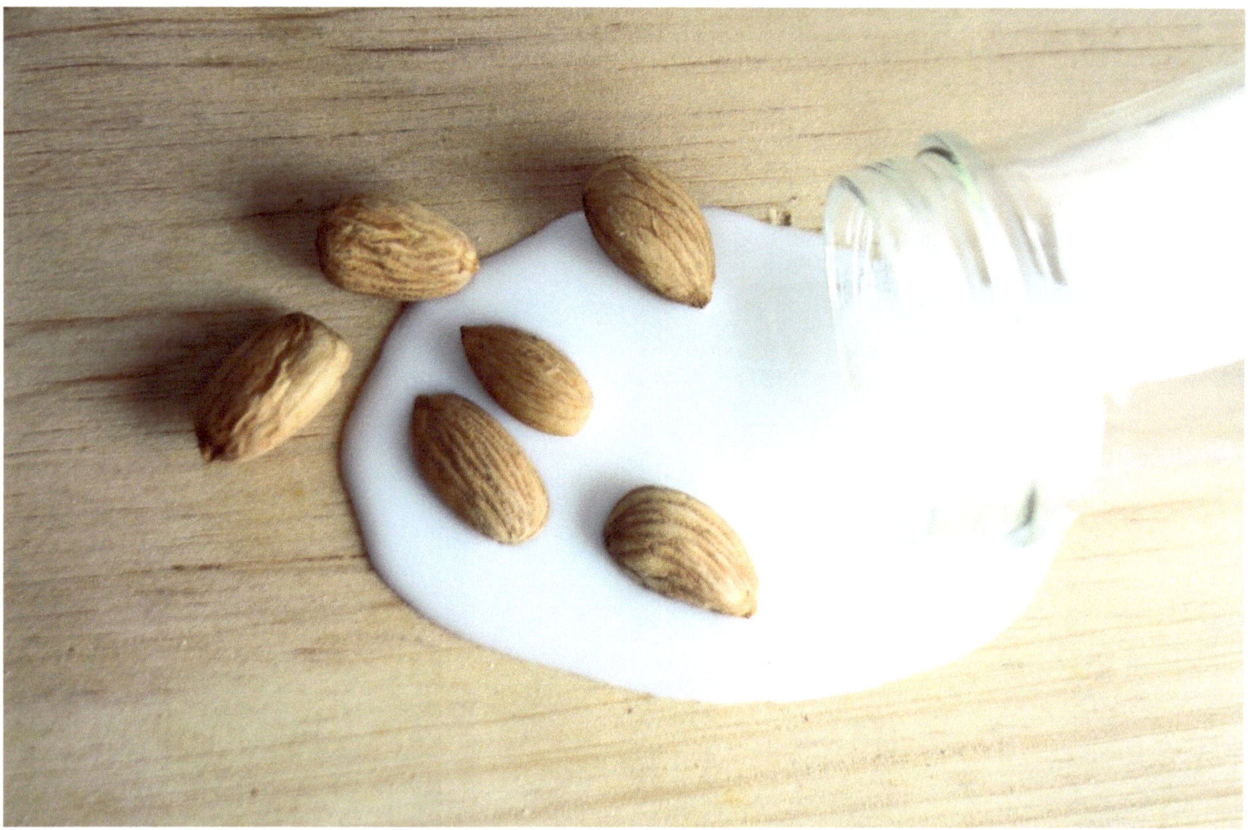

To get around the non-dairy rule, you could opt for milk alternatives, such as soya or almond milk.

Legumes

This is one you may be surprised by. Typically, legumes are considered healthy in most diets. However, if you're following the Pegan diet, you'll want to cut them out or reduce them significantly.

They can potentially cause high blood sugar, so you'll want to stick to low-starchy legumes like lentils if you want to keep them in your diet. Beans are also permitted in very small quantities due to their great fiber and protein content.

Starchy vegetables

While vegetables make up the bulk of this diet, there are still some you'll want to avoid. Starchy vegetables such as potatoes and pumpkin are advised against.

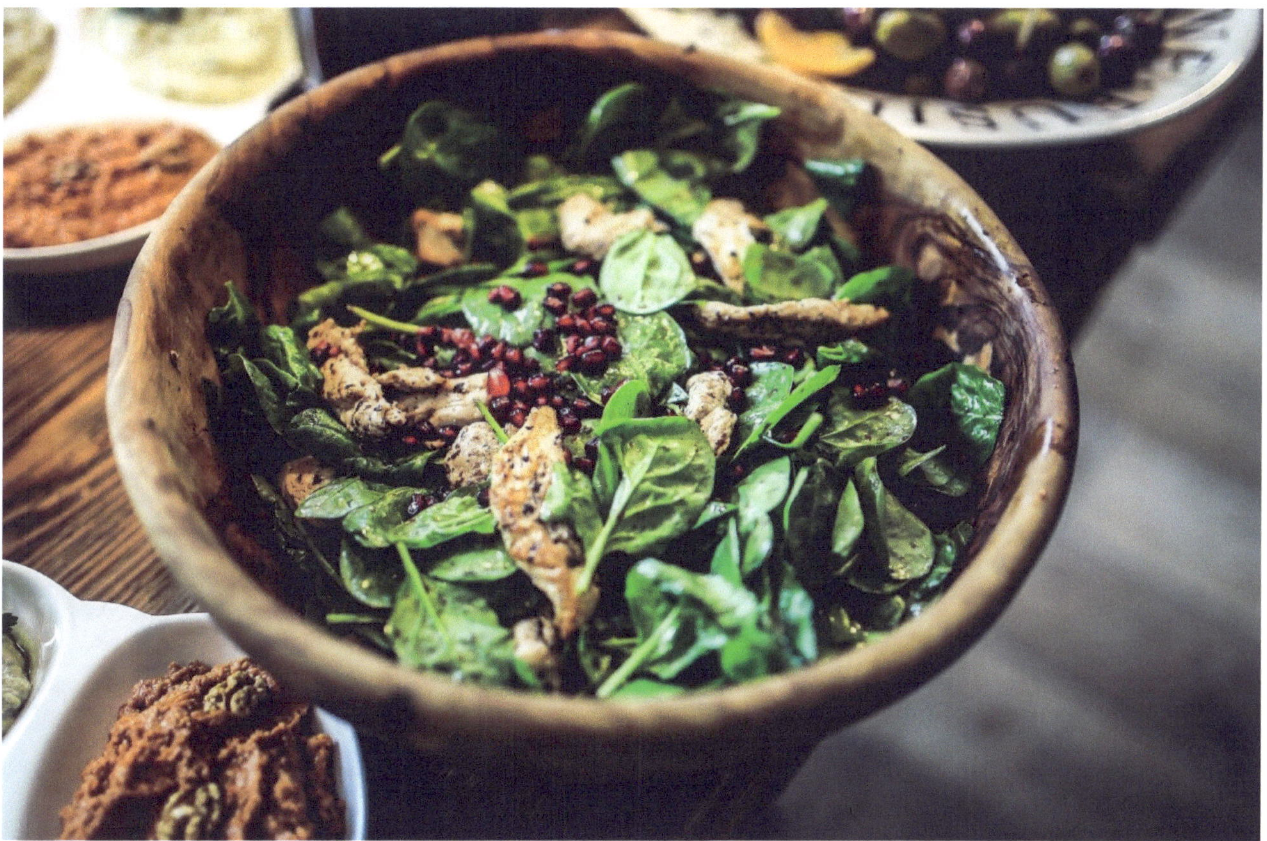

Vegetable oils

You'll find the majority of vegetable oils are prohibited too. This is because they are refined and can contain a lot of nasty ingredients. So, avoid sunflower, soybean, canola and corn oils.

Gluten and sugar

Two other things to avoid here include gluten and sugar. Keen followers of this diet avoid gluten entirely, although it is possible to consume whole gluten-free foods such as black rice and quinoa. You should just aim to eat very minimal portions.

Similarly, sugar should be cut out, or at least cut down dramatically. This is for the same reason as gluten is cut out – it can cause the sugar levels to spike. Look out for hidden sugars in foods as well as the obvious sugar ingredients.

Processed foods

Finally, you're going to want to cut out all processed foods from your diet. It has long been known that processed foods are no good for us. Instead, you want to be focusing on whole, clean foods.

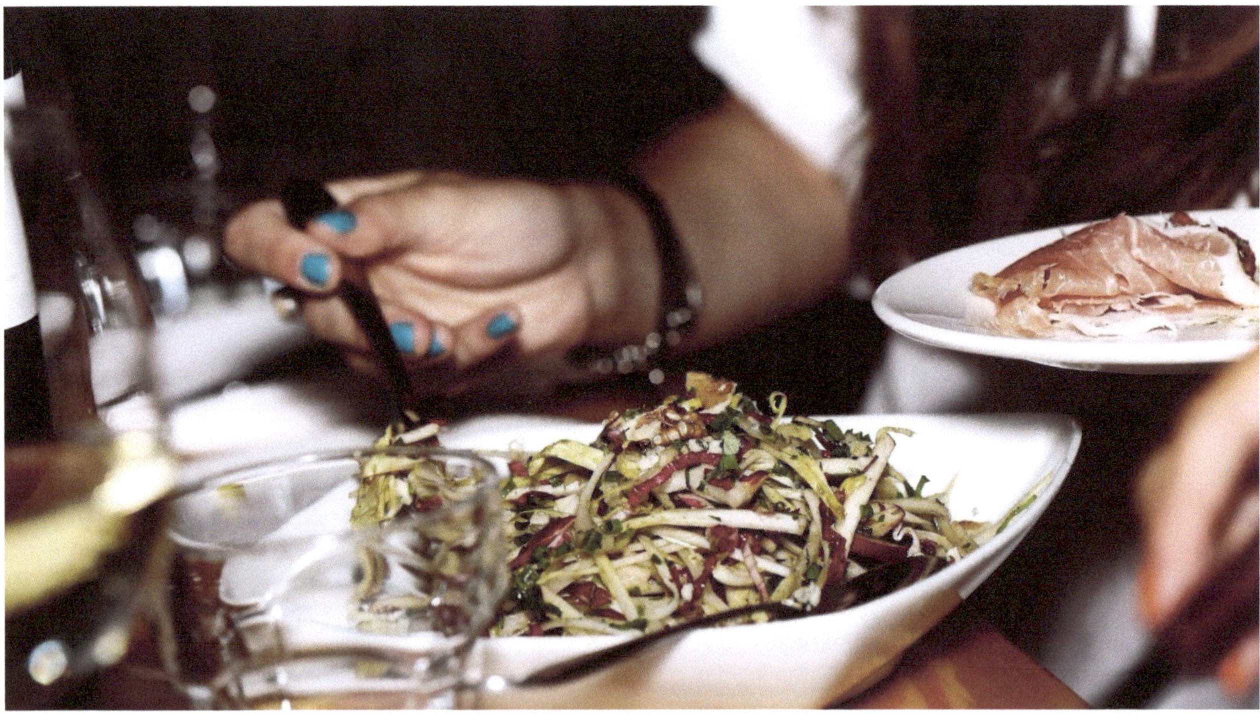

So, if you like to fill up on foods such as chips, cakes and fast food, you're going to need to undergo a dramatic change in diet. Processed foods contain a lot of bad ingredients which can be harmful to our health. If you're looking to get healthier and cut out the amount of junk you eat therefore, this diet is ideal.

While there are no strict rules in this diet, it is better to avoid the foods mentioned above. The more you follow the guidelines, the better the results you're going to experience. It's also going to be more beneficial to your health if you follow it correctly.

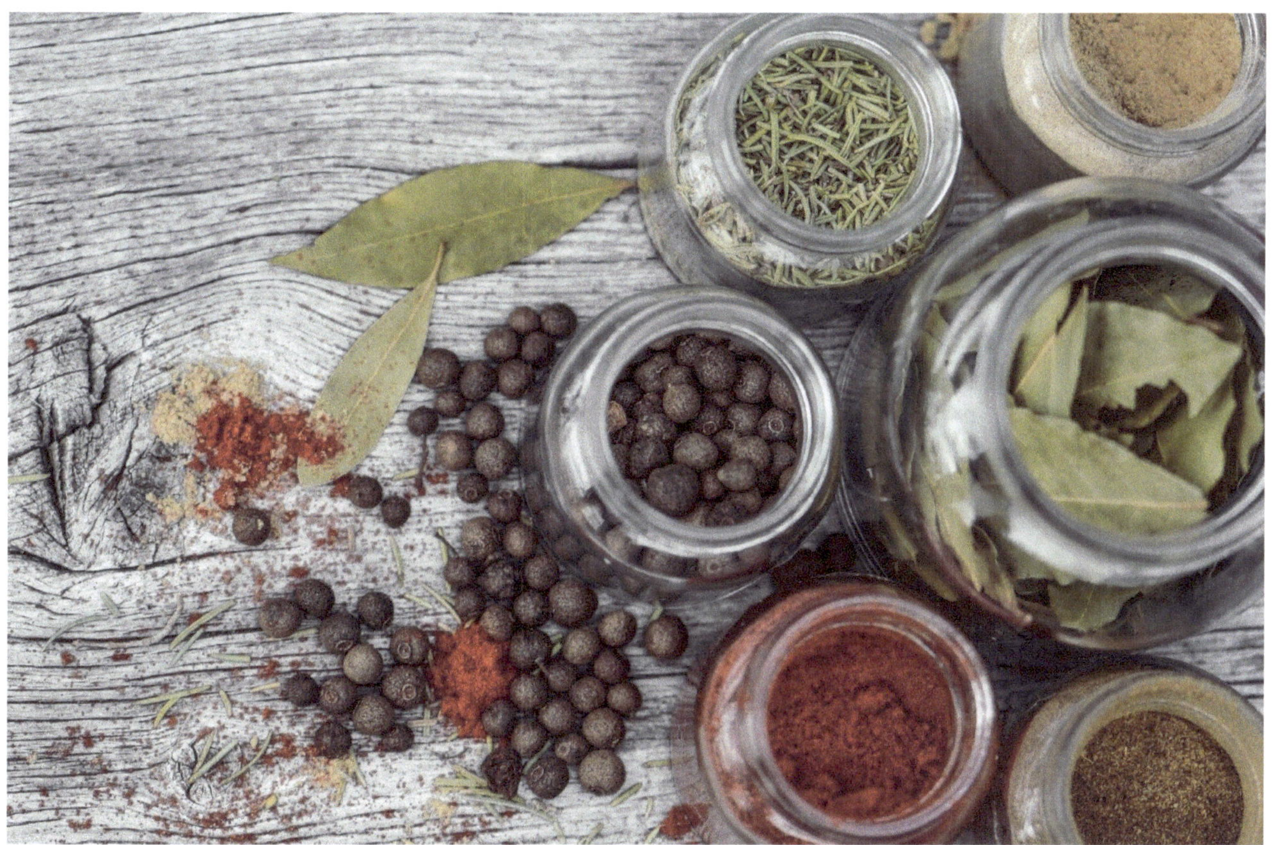

It's important to take into account what you can and can't eat on the Pegan diet in order to establish whether or not it's right for you. Limiting anything from your diet can be a challenge. However, there are ways to get around the challenges of the limited diet such as using herbs and spices to add flavor to the foods you're eating.

Benefits of the Pegan Diet

You know how it works and what you should and shouldn't eat, but what exactly are the benefits of the Pegan diet?

As it contains elements from both the paleo and vegan diets, can you expect to receive the benefits of both? Here, you'll discover the main benefits associated with Pegan diets to help you decide whether it could be the right option for you.

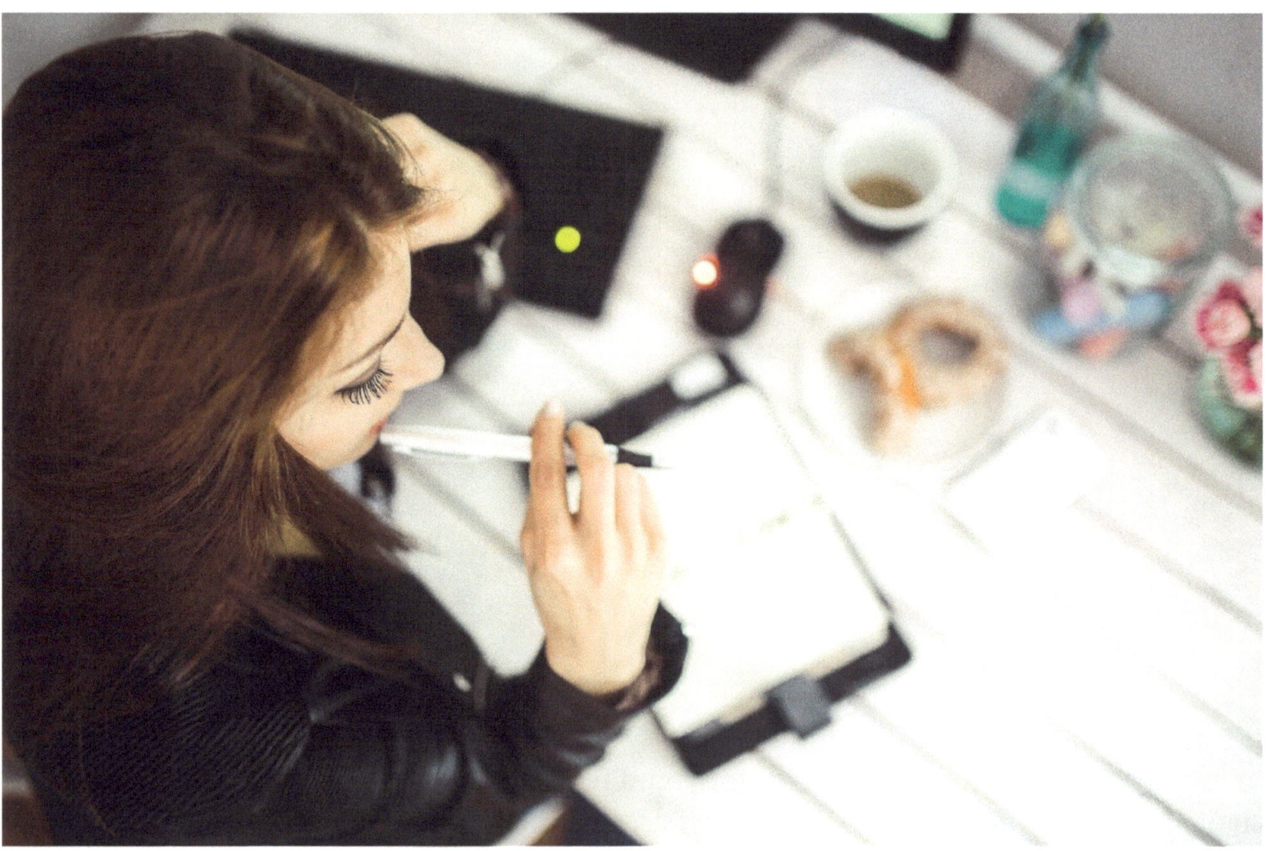

A diet rich in nutrients

The trouble with most diets which restrict what you can and can't eat, is that they often lack the nutrients you need to stay healthy. This is especially true when you're looking at the Paleo and Vegan diets by themselves.

With a vegan diet, what you can eat is significantly limited. This means the potential for nutrient deficiencies can be quite high if you aren't careful. Similarly, with the Paleo diet you'll mainly be eating meat. This means you'd miss out on the nutrients you get from other food groups.

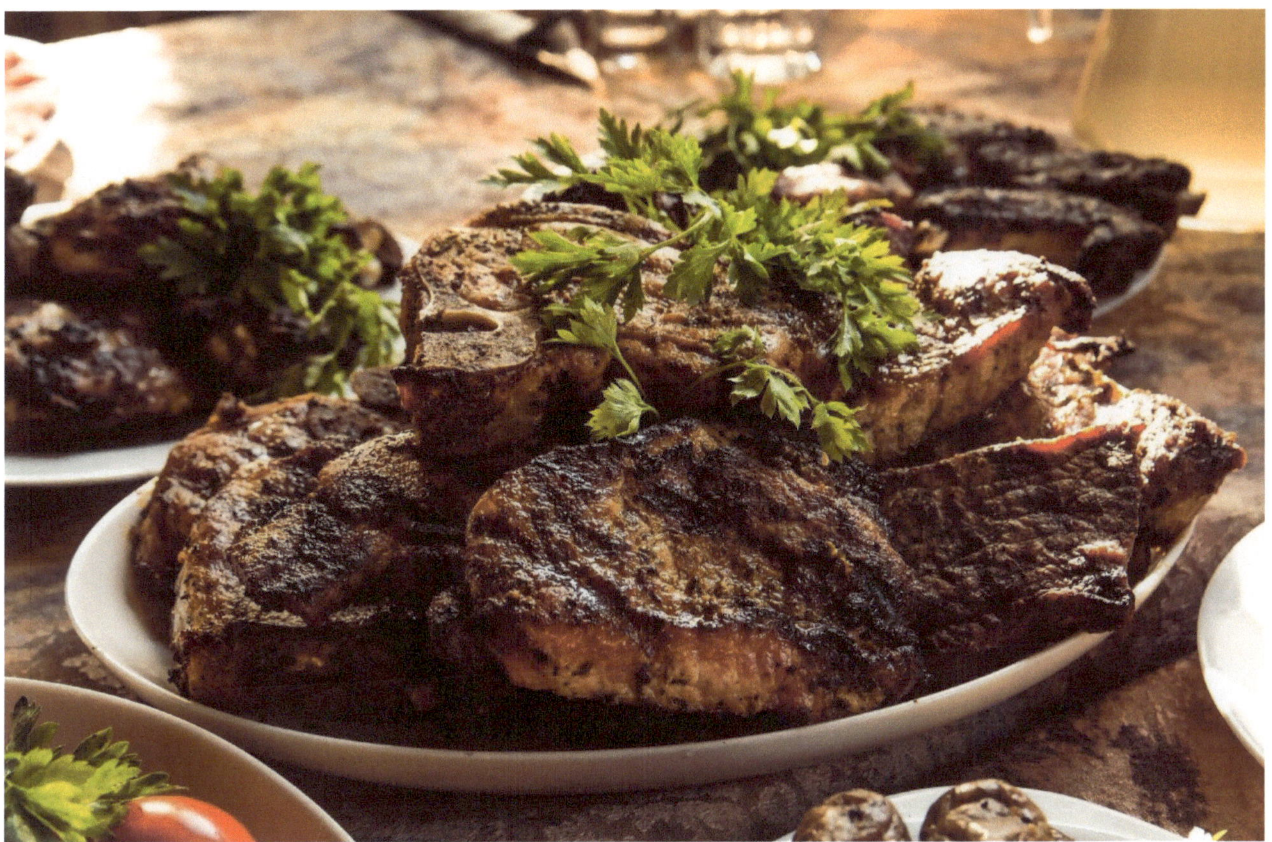

So, the fact that the Pegan diet allows both meat and plant-based foods, gives it a much higher nutritional benefit than either of the two diets alone. You'll especially be eating a high level of fruits and vegetables, which is going to keep your vitamin and mineral supplies well topped up.

Excellent for weight loss

Although the Pegan diet isn't specifically marketed for weight loss, it can help you to shed the pounds if you need to. This is because it does largely center around vegetables and plant-based foods, which typically are low in calories.

The majority of the calories you'll receive through the diet come from the vegetables. As veggies aren't exactly known for their high calorie count, you'll naturally be consuming less calories in a day than you would with many other diets. This is going to help you lose weight quickly.

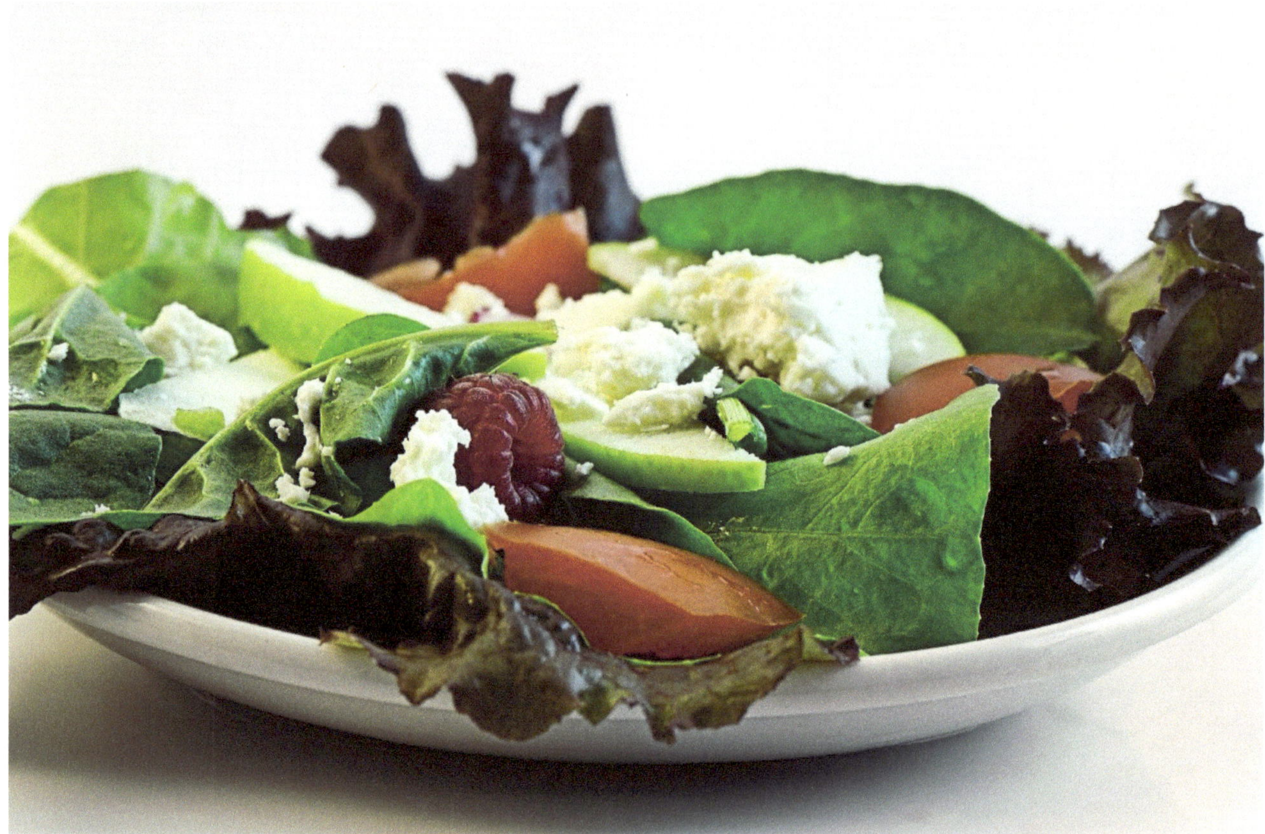

Another weight loss benefit here is that once you've lost the weight, you'll keep it off. This isn't a fad diet that you can only follow for a specific amount of time. Instead, it's more of a healthy eating lifestyle change so you'll be sustaining it potentially for the rest of your life.

Ideal for those who struggle going full vegan

Vegan diets have become extremely popular and it isn't hard to see why. However, it is one of the strictest and most restrictive diets around. Even those with the best intentions can struggle to stick to a vegan only diet. So, for those, doing the Pegan diet can be the next best thing.

Meat products are consumed in very small quantities. So, you'll get the nutrients you need from the meat, but it will take up a very small part of your daily diet. The meat you will be eating is also only coming from sustainable, locally sourced places. This means there is less chance you'll be supporting animal cruelty, which is rife in larger, commercial meat production chains.

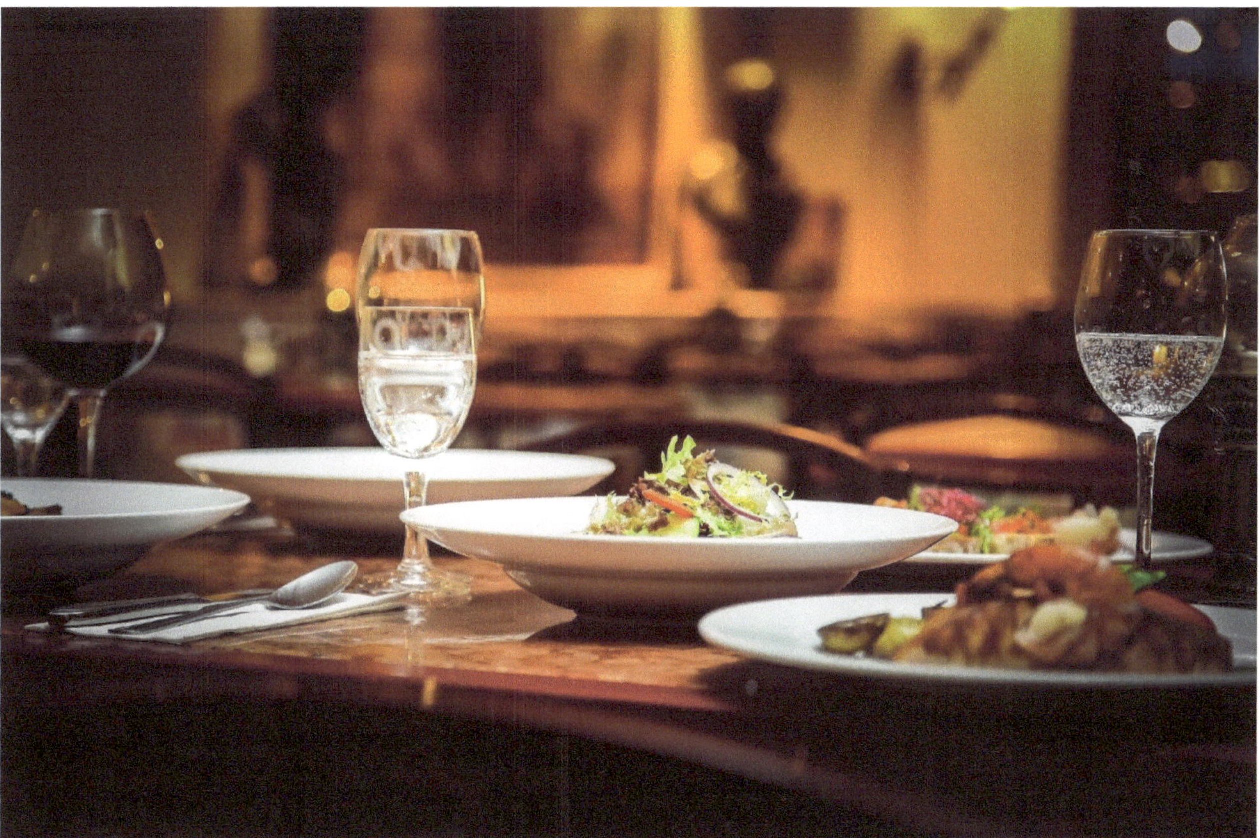

It is quite simple to follow

Although it may sound like it might be quite difficult to follow, the Pegan diet isn't overly strict. The creator recommends sticking to the guidelines 90% of the time.

The little wiggle room you're left with makes it so much easier to stick to. You won't feel like you can't have certain foods as much as you would with stricter diet plans. If you get a craving for something, you can have it as long as it's in moderation.

Ideal for those with food allergies

Finally, another great benefit of this diet is that it's great for those with food allergies. A lot of people suffer from dairy and gluten allergies. So, the fact this is a dairy and gluten free diet makes it great for those who need to be careful with their diets.

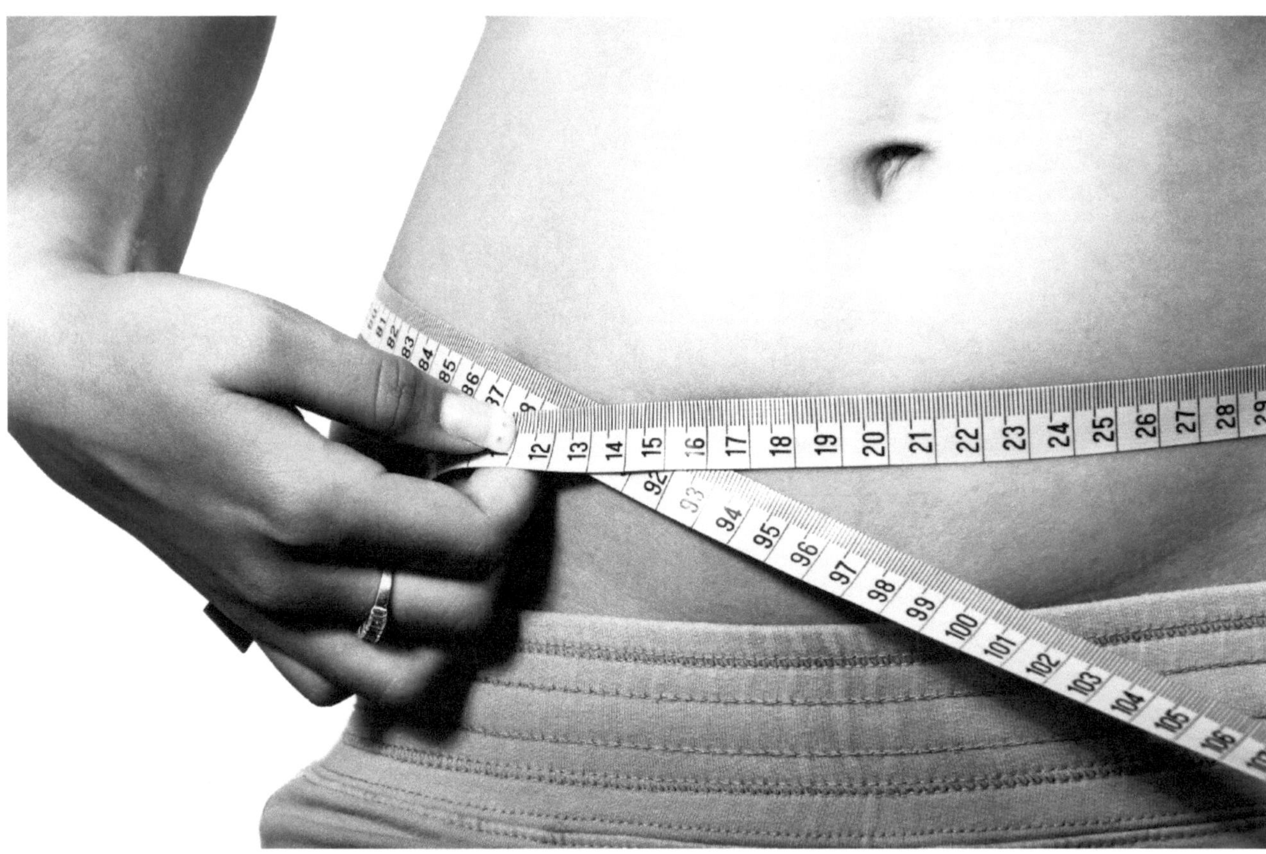

These are just a very small number of the benefits you can expect from this diet. The Pegan diet definitely isn't for everyone. However, it can be a great healthy alternative for those who struggle with the vegan or Paleo diet alone.

About the Author

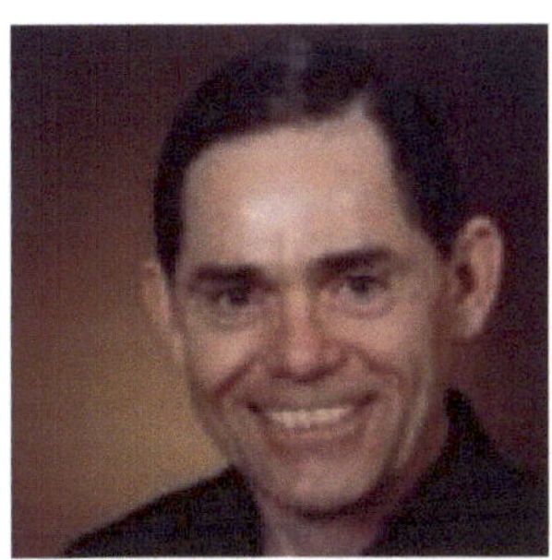

I have published numerous books on Amazon (both for Kindle and in paperback), along with other publishing platforms.

While most of my books are on health and fitness in general, I also write on baby boomer and older citizen health issues and have a recent interest in creating and printing journals/ planners and other printable products.

Besides my own writing, I also ghostwrite ebooks, books, reports, articles, blogs, autoresponder series, and do Kindle conversions for clients on a variety of topics.

Go to my website at http://ronknesswriting.com for more information or to request a quote. For a complete list of my books, go to https://www.amazon.com/Ron-Kness/e/B0072M6PYO.

Today my wife and I are retired from our careers and live in Queen Creek, AZ. I now write as a retirement business where you'll find me happily sitting in my office typing away on my laptop as I work on my next book or ghostwriting project . . . that is if we are not traveling on a cruise ship - our new-found mode of travel.